Cancer Glue for You

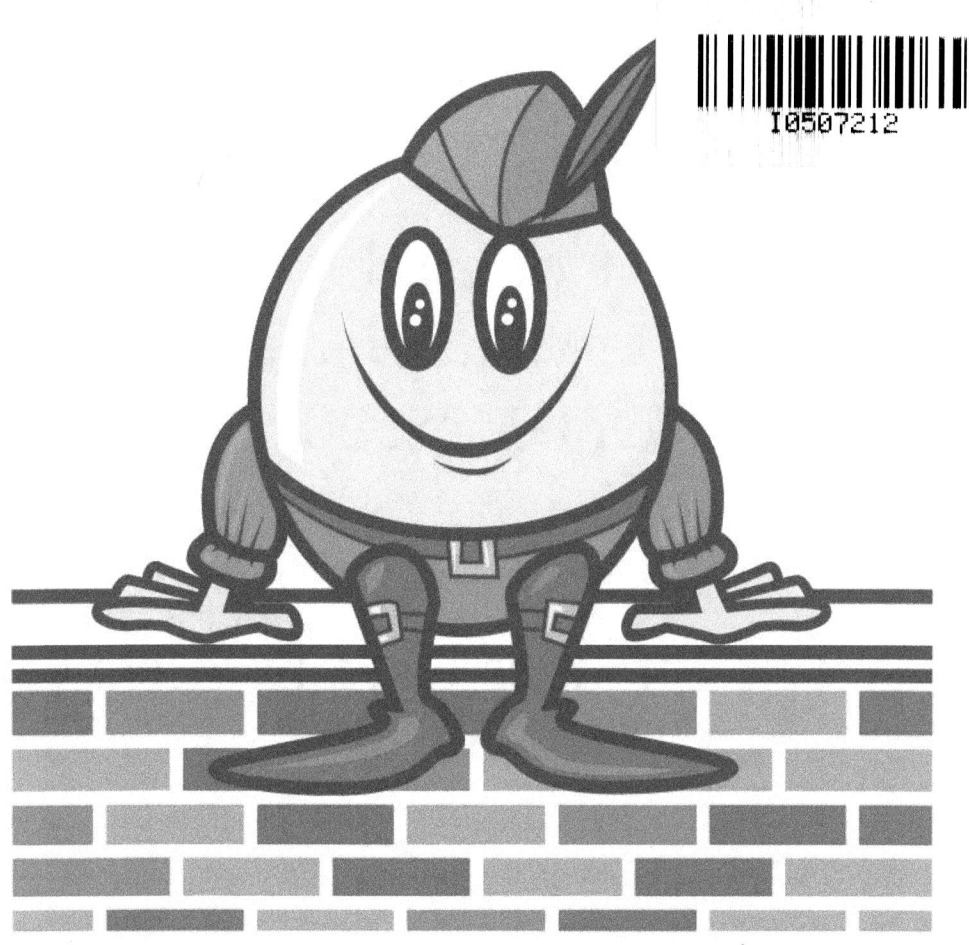

Family Energy

Reverend Mike Wanner

Copyright
Rev. Mike Wanner
October 28, 2018

Selected Images Used by License

"Healing Presents" Tab
"Prison Presents" Tab

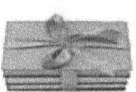

http://www.AngelRaphaelSpeaks.com

Introduction

When I was a child, my father got sick with cancer, and he had a hard time, and eventually, he was called by God, and I missed him. That was many years ago, and I wished that I could have done more for him.

I did not understand, but I wanted to, and it was impossible to know what to do to help others. I tried to comprehend but could not find answers.

The wanting to understand has influenced my life. The one thing that I remembered so firmly was the importance of kindness.

I wrote earlier about the kindness of the ambulance crews who worked with my father. In this book, I would like to talk about enhancing kindness dynamics within the family.

Each person can experience events differently so one's illness can mean different things to each person. When my father was sick, the overwhelm of uncertain circumstances made it very difficult.

Dedication

This book is dedicated to the patients being treated for cancer, and their Healing Arts care teams including all Credentialed Caregivers of Medicine, Psychological and Psychiatric Professions, Faith-based communities, Complementary Care Providers and families that have been chosen or natural.

Practitioners and Master-Teachers of the spiritual healing modalities are excellent facilitators who help to balance and soothe the active components of the emotional and mental and spiritual crises of cancer survivors. I have studied the Reiki modality and am proud to associate with the practitioners and masters.

Family members and others showing up to visit with the patient is essential, but they do not always relate well automatically.

Cancer and stress are indicators that there is still room for improvement. Each member of the family remains an independent part of the whole.

The strength of each family is about sharing and supporting each member to a varying level as determined by the ebb and flow of needs, wants, and wanting to help. Feelings of duty and must do are less helpful than the level of love that flows when one cares enough to do without being asked because they see a need, feel a call and want to offer as much as they can to help when it is needed.

The nurturing of one member of a family helps all cope.

Table of Contents

Copyright 2
Introduction 3
Dedication 4
Table of Contents 5
Disclaimer 6
1 - Why Family Matters A Lot 7
2 - Why I am Writing This Book 8
3 - Cancer is a Threat To The Whole Family 9
4 - Physical Support Includes 11
5 - Emotional Support Can Help 13
    A - Re-Integration of Families When Possible 13
    B - Constructive Thinking 14
    C - Forgiveness Can Be Energizing 15
    D - Nurturing All, Holds The Family Together 16
    E - Togetherness is Strong 17
6 - Mental Support 18
7 - Spiritual Support 20
8 - Embrace The Words of Jesus 22
9 - Cancer Prayer Suggestion 23
10 - Love is the Power 24
11 - Wrap UP! 25
12 - Thank You 26
13 - Don't Worry Ever 27
14 - Cancer Books by Rev. Mike 28
15 - Books Category Resources 29
16 - Angels Please Prayers 30
17 - Private Channeling 31
18 - Reverend Mike Wanner 32

Disclaimer

I, the author, am not involved with clinical cancer care but I have talked to many cancer patients during decades of pre-hospital ambulance care and transportation and also many years of Hospital Pastoral Care. I am sharing what is coming to me in an effort to spread understanding and trigger conversation that can be helpful. It may be that the discussion needs finessing and I invite your wisdom into the mix.

My guidance has suggested that a lot can be done to soothe the times for cancer patients and their families. I will detail my views which are not the expert positions of a Cancer Center Clinician or technician or social worker, or Medical Practitioner or Psychologist or Psychiatrist or another expert who might be helpful here.

Everything about cancer may seem very complicated, but there are always simple and practical ideas that can be embraced when a person is open to see common sense steps that are within their capability.

1 - Why Family Matters A Lot

A microcosm of the Macrocosm is the family, and the integrity of it is crucial to one's place within the universe of all that is. We cannot as individuals take in all the experiences, values and perspective of the whole universe but we can localize our attention and get enough perspective to function effectively in a complicated world.

Our family can be the reference point during times of trouble that can allow us to understand a limited perceivable base from which we can operate. We could not possibly interact with everyone out there in the world.

Our personal world of the family provides a workplace perspective balancing dynamic that operates on the record so to speak. We can be heard and what we say can be remembered.

The controlled universe also maintains any dysfunctions within the relationships as wounds that can impair functionality going forward. So, mistakes of the past insensitivities to each other can complicate future challenges by being obstructive to total commitment to the other family member's then current issue.

If one of the family has not been diligent in the care and handling or another, then open wounds may require attention before future challenges can be addressed in a helpful manner.

Old emotional wounds can be complicated and may even have contributed stress and family dis-ease to the level of intensity that may have nullified disease preventing self-healing.

2 - Why I am Writing This Book

You can read above that I have moved towards understanding and support in as many ways as I can. I write a lot about healing, and my ministry of healing messages continues to come full circle.

After taking the Our Journey of Hope Spiritual leadership training at Cancer Treatment Centers of America in Philadelphia, I became aware that the new information could integrate quite well with my lifelong learning and provide some more insight and support to others.

With this book, I would like to share ideas that may seem unusual to others but very practical to me. I also want to go one step further and add the powerful healing options of Faith, Hope, and Charity.

3 - Cancer is a Threat To The Whole Family

When Cancer hits a family, there is little opportunity for us to notice that the whole family is impacted by the challenges of the moment. During this time together, I want to share some ideas to help you know how you can deal with a Cancer Crisis in a balanced family way.

Previously I published two "Cancer Glue For Adults" books with a focus on the patient receiving love. Today let's talk about the patient remembering to give love as the giving and receiving cycle is emotional support for each member of the family and the circuit of love around brings a level of safety and vitality that does not disappoint.

In the Early days of the American pioneers, travelers needed to be concerned with attacks from bandits and animals and unfriendly circumstances. Defending each traveling wagon was enhanced by circling the wagons so there was a defense perimeter that could be clearly seen and protected.

Those inside the circle had their backs exposed only to those they knew and trusted. The safety factor allowed the encircled to focus on one attack at a time while knowing that others were defending them as they also secured the group.

The Fight against cancer is in a different direction. The cancer fight is to support the one in need so they can see that family members are turning enough attention to help but not smother them.

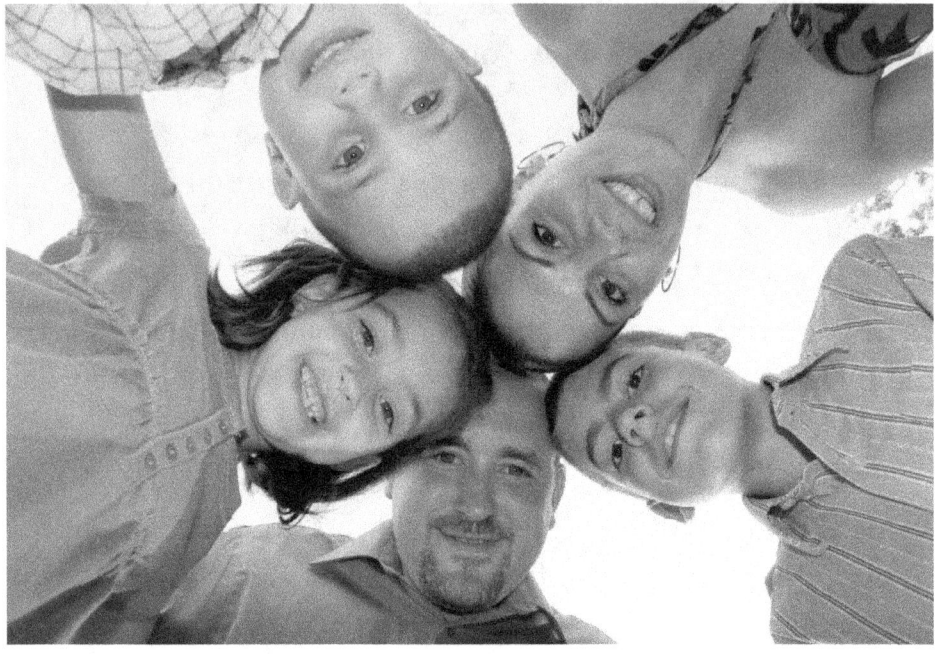

Supporting and Defending Cancer patients Has four parts:

1. Physical Support

2. Emotional Support

3. Mental support

4. Spiritual Support

4 - Physical Support Includes

Diligent Medical Care with the best Medical Devices and Brightest Human Resources available to a family's patient.

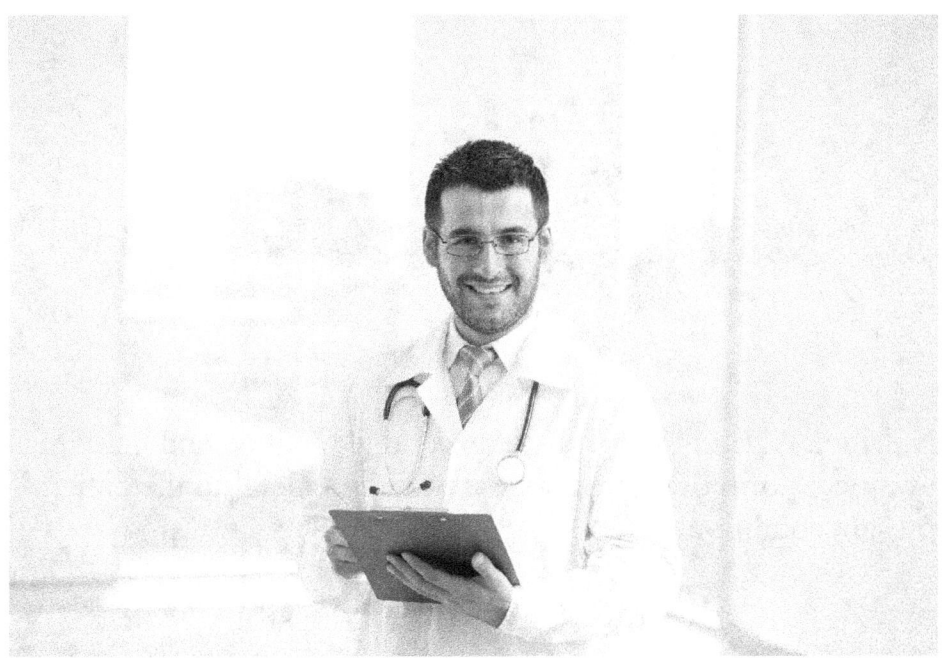

Please understand that the writer of this is a minister and is in no way able to make medical recommendations, so I defer to the Medical Professionals.

After doing a quarter century in the back of an ambulance, I know there is a lot of lying to doctors. Please do not lie to them.

Liars do not equip them with the optimal resource of complete medical history which they need to help you. They don't judge, they just evaluate, plan and treat.

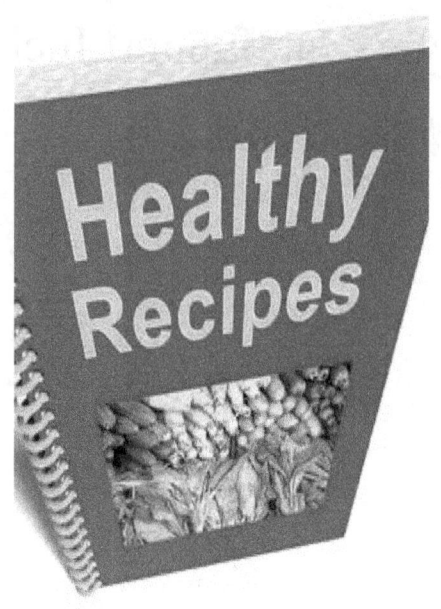

Nutrition Awareness of all that is good for healing and individual awareness of those things that are not beneficial to the patient's present condition.

Home Cooking When Possible

Old fashioned home cooking could be considered for the favorite patient in your family when the skills are available to provide them. Home cooking benefits from the love of the cook and that can help a whole lot.

Organic When Possible

Fruits and Vegetable and meats of the highest quality should be considered if available.

5 - Emotional Support Can Help

A - Re-Integration of Families When Possible
to provide a platform that can support those with Cancer

The families confronted with a family member with Cancer will get the chance to determine for themselves if they will rally around their family member or stay as cell phone centric separate identities in a co-operative but not committed world.

Emotional awareness and involvement with family members when my father was diagnosed was oriented to protect children from the realities of illness so that panic did not spread. While that was well-intentioned, for me the lack of perspective and being able to help was slightly detrimental and registered as an isolating series of events.

I had an older brother at the time and a younger Sister, My brother was 17 in denial and soothed himself separately from the family. My sister was 7 and leaned on me for perspective and comfort. I was eleven and overwhelmed with it all.

I did not feel that I was empowered at that time and my craving for understanding is brought full circle now.

B - Constructive Thinking

Every Family is different and finding the love for the foundation of family support you think is wise can be a challenge so you just might need a plan. In your family, you might be the only one who is not the patient, and that can make it hard but old wounds may need to be addressed for healing to happen.

It can be effortless to surrender to the complexity of some situations and sometimes even necessary to do so. Planning can optimize possibilities, so please consider it.

Identifying some sore spots/issues between family members can be a place to start. Prayer for guidance can be an excellent second step. Reality checks and discussions can follow, as can reconnections.

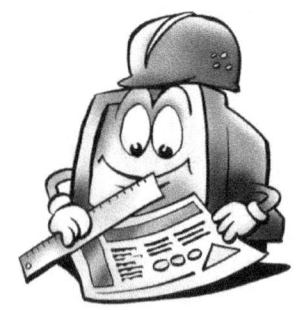

C - Forgiveness Can Be Energizing

Resentment can last a long time and negativity held too long may be unhealthy if it results in a lessening of life force to help healing when it is needed. Humans are subtle beings, and their energies with subtle energy fields can be impacted in subtle ways.

The movie, "What the Bleep do we Know" contained a segment about water crystals and the work of Dr. Emoto in his book "The Hidden Messages in Water." Dr. Emoto's book shows identical water samples from one source which were treated exactly the same except for the exposure of one to subtle energy through prayer or positive words.

He would later take drops from each sample and freeze them and slice them and put them on slides under a high powered microscope and photograph the slides. The photos showed formation that was dramatically different.

Those exposed to positive energy were beautiful crystalline formation where the other was less attractive and some even like bad mutations.

Emotions within families can run the scale from Love to Hate. Sometimes the trigger of the feeling could be an issue on a level of potential between the highly positive value and the profoundly negative one. While we are each mostly water like the crystals above, reverting to positivity seems a logical approach to more balanced and peaceful relationships. Forgiveness is effective at releasing negativity for all.

D - Nurturing All, Holds The Family Together

Even agreeing to disagree, can be a resolution to old wounds and victimizations. Families reaching a point of accommodation can encircle all perspectives in a new understanding to keep bad things out and optimal love within.

Embracing the crisis with the love and support of your family goes a long way to reduce stress and bring faith, hope, charity, and healing.

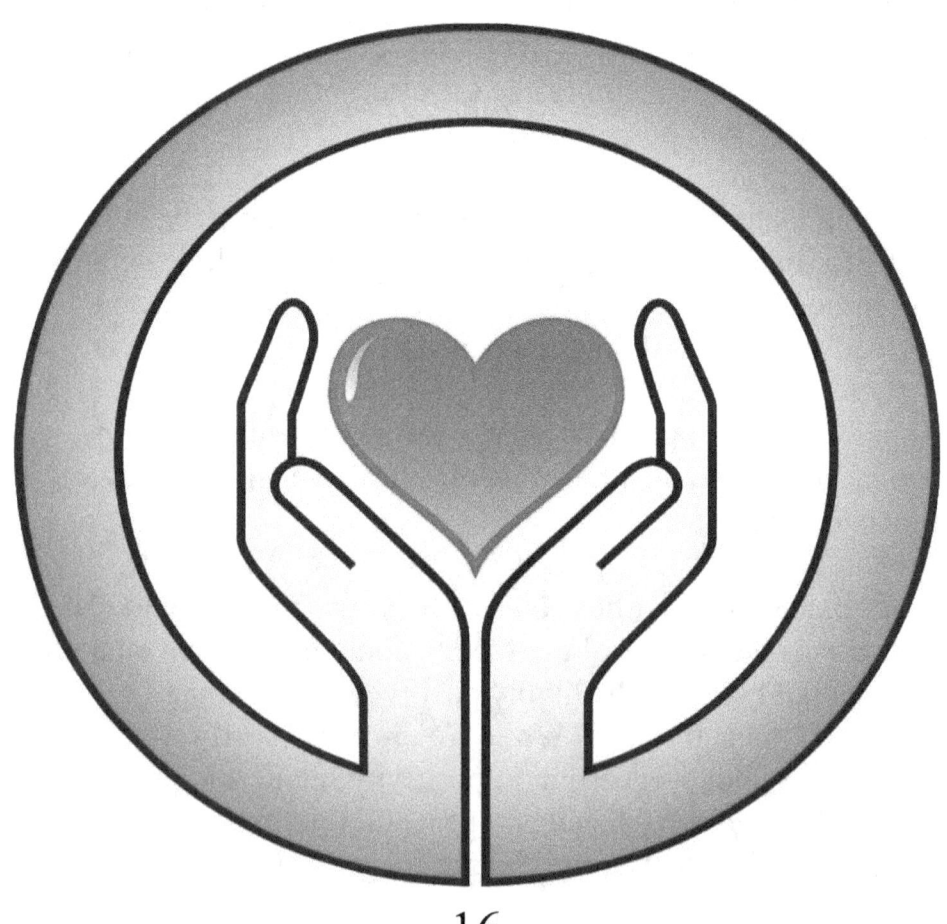

E - Togetherness is Strong

Improved Understanding and balance in families can strengthen the foundation for healing. Adding concrete to a sand mix builds stability, like filling and sharing your heart full of love with the whole family.

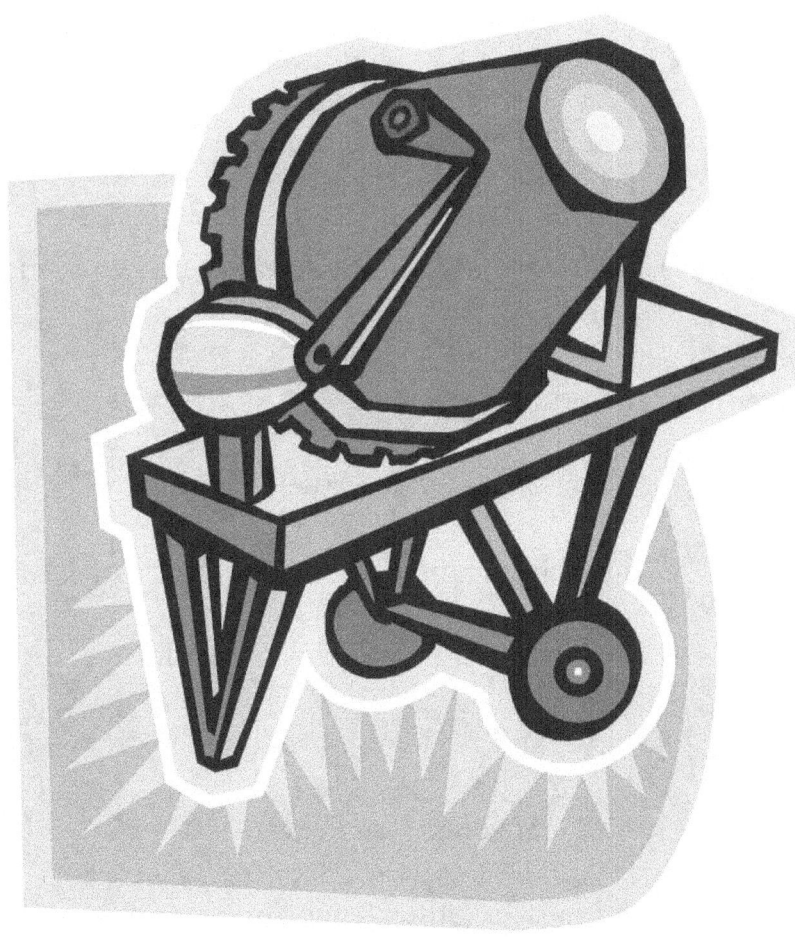

6 - Mental Support

Consider Adding Family, Wise Friends, and Associates To Your Physical Support and Emotional Support

Medical Support is the key to Physical Healing optimization,

Emotional Support is the key to Optimized Emotional Stability.

Knowing You Have Medical and Emotional Support is the key to Physical, Emotion and Mental Healing.

When Cancer is present, those with it need to move towards all that Can Be!

Information Shares the Power Potentials!

Action Activates Potential!

Embracing Family brings strength!

Invite Your Tribe into Your Struggle!

Unity Can Provide More Strength!

Persistence Can Prevail!

Action is Healthier Than Anxiety.

Whatever is going on in the head of a cancer patient can influence everything within the person. If the patient is you or a loved one, clear thinking can help.

The simple act of taking the time to talk or listen or respectfully disagree can bring peace. The critical part is the that the conversation carries the emotion and when the feeling moves in the flow then any toxicity of thought has an exit path and the discharge is able to destress much more than the mind.

When clear thinking is added to all the medical support and nutritional support with good cooking and the best food, and we add to that all the emotional support of family and the community all in healed alignment, and we combine clear thinking then we are moving in a triple support way towards an optimal situation.

The triple support spectrum can efficiently enliven the one who has been in treatment so struggle can be less and efficient use of the energy available in each of the three areas is as close to vibrancy as possible.

7 - Spiritual Support

You are the creation of the God Most High who has brought you to life for a Divine purpose. You were brought here by the love of your creator to do something Divine.

You may or may not know why you are here. The lover of you is the Supreme Source of that knowledge.

Your journey may not have gone as well as the Divine plan, and there is no need to worry about all that. The simple fact that you are still here has a message for you and the rest of us.

You may feel that your life is upside down. Maybe things were being done in the wrong order, and you now have a chance to reset your priorities.

Regardless of what has gone before, you have more life remaining that can be spent in the study of and the development of potential resources. Can you seek the bigger picture of life and health and healing?

Your Auto-Pilot may need to be reset. Many people go through life with the settings and belief systems that were installed naturally by Divine Order or unnaturally by the best intentions of loving people who may not have been in the optimal position to choose wisely at the time.

Everything can change over time, and if you are still on autopilot and the settings have not been reviewed and evaluated lately, then it may be time to do that. When you go to your doctor, he will likely take your vital signs to see if anything has changed recently. You can check your settings.

Earlier I wrote a book called *Reiki Help For Cancer Care In Pottstown, Pa,* and the book was about how the Spiritual Healing Technique called Reiki helped my friend. The clinical care there included it, and that helped her.

As she sat there and watched others, she noticed those who were weakest and intended Reiki energy go to them if they were subconsciously willing to receive it and she also prayed for them to raise their vibration even if they did not accept the Reiki.

Like the doctors, you can be checking for changes and adjustments that could help keep you or your loved one up to date and in optimal balance in all areas of your life.

When Cancer is present, those with it could feel sorry for themselves and allow the energy as is or they can be pro-active and bless themselves and others with positive thoughts and actions. Giving to others is like receiving yourself as you change the focus from not enough joy to plenty to share.

Joy Is A Natural Byproduct of Faith!

Unity of Your support systems Can Provide Strength to pull yourself together!

8 - Embrace The Words of Jesus

Jesus declared that the work that he does, you can also do if you believe in him.

John 14.10 "…I speak not of myself: but the father that dwelleth in me, he doeth the works. "

John 14.12 "…I say unto you, He that believeth on me, the works that I do shall he do also: and greater works than these shall he do; because I go unto my father."

John 14.18 "I will not leave you comfortless: I will come to you."

Mark 9:23 " …all things are possible to him that believeth."

Cancer patients can enhance their healing by taking a break from focusing on themselves and look across the aisle at the others and bless them in any way that seems right. You can be blessed as you bless others with thoughts, prayers, blessings, and energy.

9 - Cancer Prayer Suggestion

Mother God
Father God
Almighty God
God Of Healing
God Of Light
God of Joy

I/We Recognize You.

I/We open to Unify With You.

I/We Claim healing for Cancer for all as we unify and love you and all people of all religions & all skin colors & all nations & all beings & all species & all that is.

As I/we claim healing and share love, I/we see the healing manifest for all.

I/We Acknowledge your joy, love, compassion, understanding and the healing now.

Thank You, God,
AND SO IT IS!

10 - Love is the Power Of God

Love

Is

The

Power

Of

God

Invite God To Smile
By
Giving God's Love To ALL!

You Lose Nothing
&
Gain Everything!

11 - Wrap UP!

I have been doing pastoral visitation for the last fourteen years at the Jefferson - Frankford Hospital in Philadelphia, and I have seen a lot of things, and am still amazed at the Power of Belief and Intention.

What You Say Is Your Truth!

Say the Right Thing To Yourself
And You Succeed

Say the Wrong Thing To Yourself
And You Fail

Change Wrong Words To Right & Succeed

You Can Be Awesome When You Tune Your Conscious Focus

(Laser Sharp R U)

**May All Who Read This Be Blessed
AND SO IT IS!**

Rev. Mike

12 - Thank You

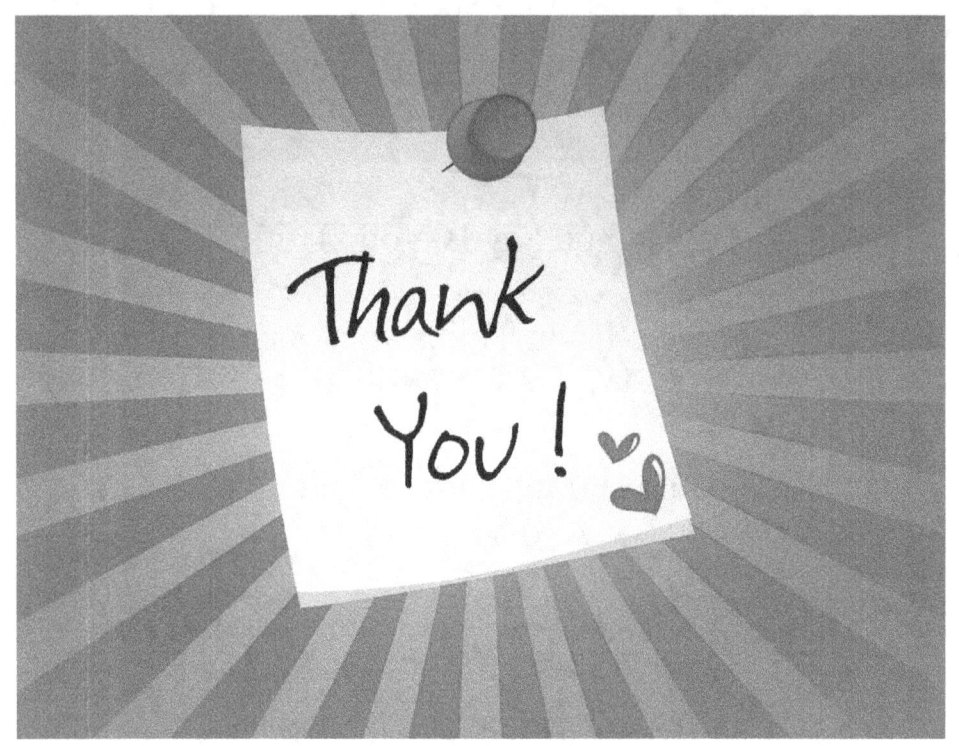

For
Considering
These
Ideas

13 - Don't Worry Ever

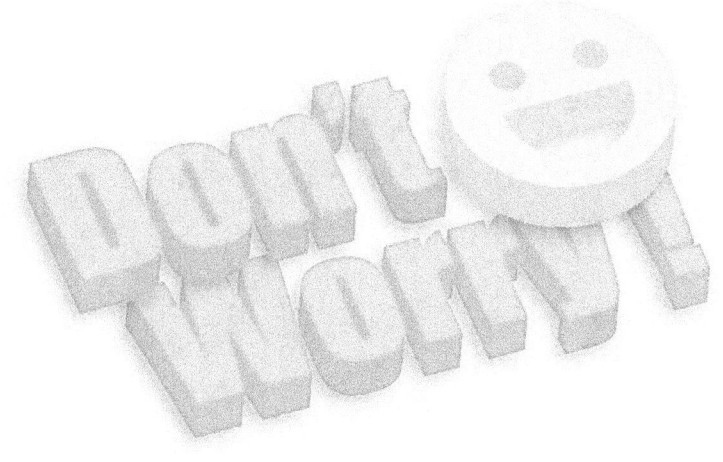

Ever

It Does Not Help Prayer Still Does!

Resource: http://Create-A-Prayer.com

14 - Cancer Books by Rev. Mike

Cancer Glue For Adults: Love From Reiki
http://amzn.com/B07JQPBWW6

Cancer Glue For Adults: Love From Kids
http://amzn.com/B00MS6M77I

Does Reiki Love Heal Cancer?: Transcribed True Stories Of Spiritual Healing
http://amzn.com/B00MS6M77I

Reiki Help For Cancer Care in Pottstown, PA: Cecilia Appreciates PMMC Cancer Center
http://amzn.com/B071XBTSFX

Reiki For Cancer
http://amzn.com/B07873YKLJ

15 - Books Category Resources
at www.Amazon.com

Distant Healing (or Mail List) e-mail mikewann@voicenet.com

Veterans Healing Six Pack plus 2
http://angelraphaelspeaks.com/healing-books/veterans/

PTSD Power Pack
http://angelraphaelspeaks.com/healing-books/ptsd/

Angel Raphael Speaks Series & Other Angel Books
http://angelraphaelspeaks.com/

Reiki
http://angelraphaelspeaks.com/healing-books/reiki/

Children
http://angelraphaelspeaks.com/healing-books/children/

Emergency Medical Kindness
http://angelraphaelspeaks.com/healing-books/emergency-medical-kindness/

Cancer
http://angelraphaelspeaks.com/healing-books/cancer/

Addictions
http://angelraphaelspeaks.com/healing-books/addictions/

Miscellaneous Healing
http://angelraphaelspeaks.com/healing-books/misc-healing/

Prison Books - 50+ Prison Books
http://angelraphaelspeaks.com/prison-books/

16 - Angels Please Prayers

Addict's
Angels of Healing Selected
Help Me to Stay Directed
Come To Me From The Sky
I Am Ready to Succeed Not Try
If I Don't Invite You In
I Might Not Win
I Have Been Lost For Too Long
Help Me To Stay Strong

Alcoholic's
Angels of Healing On High
Help Me to Stay Dry
Come To Me From The Sky
I Am Ready to Succeed Not Try
If I Don't Invite You In
I Might Not Win
I Have Been Lost For Too Long
Help Me To Stay Strong

Prayers Above From

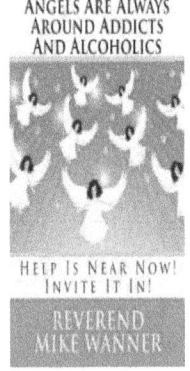

http://AngelRaphaelSpeaks.com/AAAAAAA/
The Link Above Has the Core Messages from the book on drop-down pages.

17 - Private Channeling

Angel Raphael Speaks a series of free messages that are channeled through Reverend Mike Wanner for the Highest good and Highest Healing of all concerned.

Many questions arise about Reverend Mike doing private channeling, and he does help with that so E-mail him.

Reverend Mike is available worldwide as a psychic channel, emotional release facilitator, spiritual energy practitioner & teacher, and public speaker.

He looks forward to meeting you soon! Email - mikewann@voicenet.com 215-342-1270

PRIVATE SPIRITUAL READINGS/channelings or Spiritual Healing Sessions: Telephone or in person.

Rev. Mike is available for individual, intuitive one-on-one sessions with you, his Guide Family, and your Guides. He helps by offering clarity on emotional situations about your life, your purpose, your spirituality, and your release of stuffed emotions and cellular memory.

Connect to the love of your Guides today!

For more information, Please visit

http://angelraphaelspeaks.com/channel/

18 - Reverend Mike Wanner

Rev. Mike Wanner started his spiritual and ministerial studies with Reiki in 1993 and had studied seven styles of Reiki in the U.S., Japan, Canada, Denmark, and Australia. He is certified to teach.

He became certified to teach Integrated Energy Therapy in 1999 and co-taught the first IET class of the new Millennium. Mike began dowsing in 2001.

Ordained as an Interfaith Minister of the Circle of Miracles Ministry and a Metaphysical Minister of the International Metaphysical Ministry, Rev. Mike practices and teaches spiritual energy therapies in the Philadelphia Area.

Rev. Mike holds ministerial degrees from the University of Metaphysics and the University of Sedona. He is a Pastoral Care Associate at Jefferson - Frankford Hospital. He taught at the National Academy of Massage Therapy and Health Sciences.

Rev. Mike was a faculty member of the Medical Mission Sister's Center for Human Integration's School of Integrated Body/Mind Therapies in Fox Chase, Philadelphia, PA for twelve years.

For a complete Biography, Please visit

http://ReverendMikeWanner.com/Bio